Detox While You Eat (6 + 8)

A Simplified Whole Body Detox and Allergy Cleanse Program

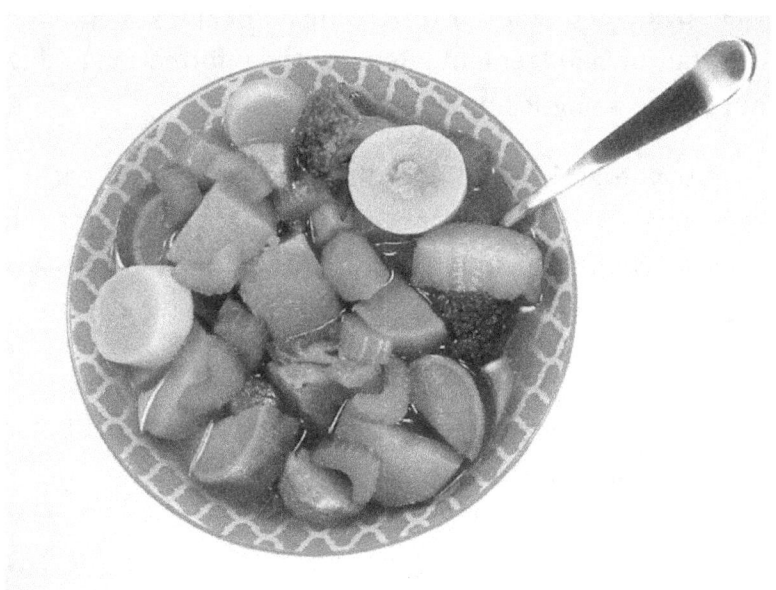

By Dr. Jacqueline Grooms, D.C.

Contents

THE SIMPLIFIED PROGRAM 27

Preface

14 Weeks – What??!! Yes, you will have to do the work to get the best results. It will take time to flush your system and keep the toxins out long enough to begin really healing. The program takes you safely through 6 weeks of detox plus 8 weeks of food reintroduction for determining food allergies. It is doable because while it limits the types of foods you eat; it doesn't limit the amount. You can eat what you want and how much you want within the parameters of the program.

The program works with your body's natural detoxification system so you don't change your body chemistry or harm yourself. It also doesn't require you to restrict yourself to one specific food. That's extremely unhealthy. Short term programs that give you short term results can have long term consequences. You don't want fast changes by consuming a diet that can't be maintained. This could slow your metabolism or cause chemical imbalances. This book takes you through a slow process where you come out healthier and with healthier habits in the end.

It is also a simple read. I didn't include all the science or any filler information such as meal plans or pages and pages of recipes you won't ever use. It is just the program. The science is easy to find with simple searches if you would like more, and you can check out my website for additional tips.

For more information, visit my website at **Nutri4.com**.

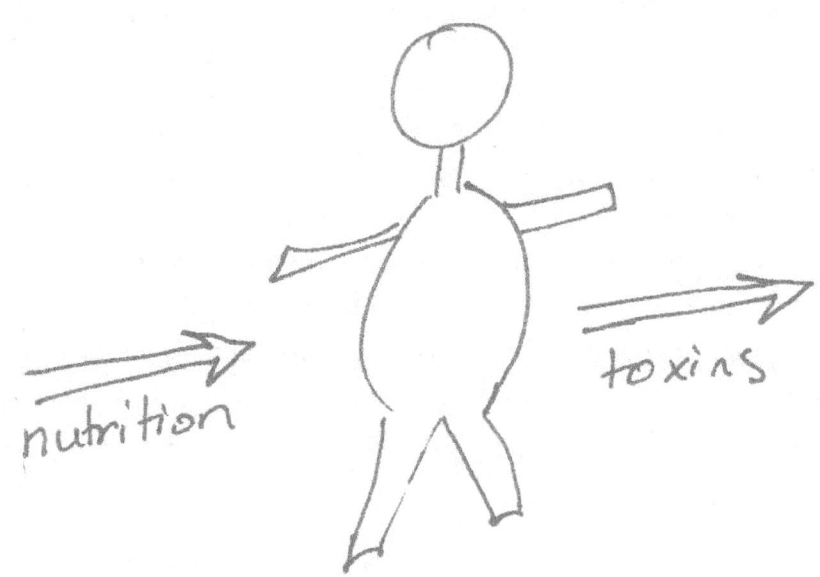

Choosing Yourself

"I am so tired!"

Ever say that? Do you crawl out of bed in the morning already exhausted? Do you aim for your couch as soon as you can make it home from work? Do you make excuses to friends when they want to go out?

This is the number one indicator that your health is lousy. Yes, there are symptoms galore - constipation, joint pain, headaches, allergies, bloating, reflux, high cholesterol, high blood pressure, hormone imbalance, and the list goes on and on. Your body can cry out for help with all kinds of different symptoms, but at the base of it your body is working like crazy to heal itself which takes lots of energy. When your body is working so hard to survive, there isn't any energy left for you to enjoy life.

Why? There are combinations of different factors. First, genetics and illnesses are things you are born with. These are luck of the draw and you just have to live and compensate for them. Sounds harsh, but they are not factors we can control, so let's focus on what we can control. There are thousands of health books out there, dozens of health programs, TV shows dedicated to health, doctors specializing in nutrition, stores and products targeting health and yet most Americans are still depressingly unhealthy.

Let's start with a basic premise: YOU ARE IN CHARGE OF YOUR OWN HEALTH. Doctors and health insurance are for when you get in trouble and need help with the cleanup. Striving for health is your responsibility alone and takes a lot of work.

Step One: DECIDE TO CHANGE

Yep, the hardest thing to do when trying to get healthy is changing your lifestyle. It is easy to say "eat right and exercise", but when you are exhausted just getting up to find the remote, cooking and moving are the last things you want to think about. This is the big catch 22 when it comes to health, you know what to do because the information is everywhere, you just don't have the energy to do it.

Well, suck it up. The first step is to just force yourself to start. I tend to be an all-or-nothing person. I am either on a "diet" or not. When I am, I eat right. When I am not, I go through the drive through or crack open a box. The only "veg-ing" I do is on my couch. I know my weaknesses, so it is time to find my strengths.

Step Two: MAKE THE CHANGE

Start this program right now. Don't plan it for after the holidays or even next week. Just commit yourself to getting healthy and start right now. Procrastination will only reinforce established bad habits. Just – Do – It!

Step Three: KEEP IT UP

At the end of this program, you will have established new and healthier eating habits. It is up to you to continue them. You have already proved to yourself that you can do it, so give yourself credit for taking charge of your own health. When you start to revert back, and you will, just come back to the lessons you learned during this program and get back on track.

Why This Program Works

Easy On Your Body

Instead of putting your body into shock with extreme dietary limits or changes, this program is focused on adding nutrition. While you will eliminate foods from your diet, you will do so at a gradual pace. This keeps the body from going into shock where chemical and metabolic changes can cause more harm than good. It also slows toxin release so your body can more easily remove them rather than trying to store them again or shocking your system.

This shock to the body can cause liver damage, kidney damage, and even acne as your body tries to push toxins out at a rate it can't handle. You may also feel faint from insulin imbalance, get foggy brain, nausea, and stomach issues. Your metabolism will also be affected where you might lose a few pounds in the beginning, but you end up with a lower set point which causes weight gain when you go back to eating normally.

No Products to Buy

You may want to add supplements to fortify organs and aid repair, but these are optional. This is what detox products do. They simply give your body additional nutrients. However, you can also get the same results with a more gradual program. You will already add nutrients to your body by simply following the diet so the choice for more is yours.

I like supplements. In fact, I use and recommend them often. They are great for addressing specific imbalances or deficiencies, but should be used to aid, not replace eating your nutrients. If you do choose to use them, make sure they are food based and do not contain harmful fillers or binders.

Find Your Food Allergies

This program has you eliminate particular groups of foods over time. Then, once your body is flushed out, you will start to add foods back in. If you have a food allergy or food sensitivity your will notice immediately when you add them back. You will know by getting stomach issues, acne, feeling sluggish, or other easily noticed symptoms. We are so used to feeling bad that we don't notice many of the reactions our bodies have to food. We also can't always tell which foods make us feel bad. By eliminating many of the usual culprits and then adding them back slowly, we can discover how food affects us.

Toxins, Energy, and Weight Loss

The main purpose of this program is to reduce toxins in our bodies to help us feel better. By giving your body a break from the onslaught of bad food choices, you give it a chance to clean out and start healing. This healing will take a long time, far beyond the parameters of the program. This just jump starts it and you need to maintain healthy eating for the healing to complete its process. This process is dependent on the current health of your body. The longer and worse your diet has been and/or the longer you have been ill means the more healing to be done. If you have been harming your body for years, it could be months on the maintenance portion for you. If you already eat healthy and have few problems, you probably already eat the maintenance recommended diet so this will just be a "spring cleaning" for you.

As you heal, your energy should return. You will start feeling better, thinking clearer and feel like getting out more. This increased energy will get you up and moving which will just help you heal all the faster.

As for weight loss, well that isn't the point of this program, but if you have bad eating habits, then eating right will naturally help the weight come off. The biggest benefit for weight loss I have found is the increased energy I spoke of above that helps you want to get up and out. You will probably feel like walking more or even adding exercise to your day. You will feel better and want to keep eating right which means your weight may continue to come off if needed. Again, if you already eat right and exercise then you probably won't see a large reduction, but for those who need this program the most will probably see 5-20 lbs. or even more come off.

Why Is It A 14 Week Program Rather Than A 3 Day, 5 Day, 10 Day, or even 21 Day?

There are so many options out there, so why go so slow? Can't I just eliminate everything the first week? The problem is the body's reaction to toxin release. Some chemicals take longer to be eliminated, such as caffeine and sugar. They also need to be out of your system longer for your body to stop craving them. If you take medications, eliminating foods changes your chemical makeup and you will need to watch how it affects you and your meds. You also don't want your body going into shock and kicking in other chemical processes. This can slow your metabolism, cause digestive issues, or other undesirable effects. Give your body time to adjust to each stage.

Since it is also about feeding your body nutrients, it takes time for your gut to repair and start absorbing nutrients effectively again. You need this time to heal, and since you can eat all the vegetables you want, 14 weeks really shouldn't be an issue. Just make this time for yourself.

Exercise

Exercise is a vital part of healing. Your toxic build-up needs to be removed and exercise aids in that process. Getting your heart pumping doesn't just build muscle and stamina, but the oxygen and pumping blood carries toxins through your filtering system (liver and kidneys). Sweat also carries toxins out through your skin. This is one reason why people may feel better after exercise. Another benefit is that it reduces stress which takes energy and healing away from other issues.

How much? Well how much do you already do? If you already have a routine, then yay, keep it up. If not, then get off the couch and move. Take a walk and enjoy the fresh air. Take the stairs. If nothing else, stand in front of the TV and stretch and walk in place while you are watching your favorite show. Just move. Sitting all day will kill you. It will hamper the body's ability to remove toxins and allow build up that will eventually let diseases develop. Movement is life.

What You Need for The Program

Overview of The Program

You will add good foods while slowly eliminating foods that may cause sensitivity. Then you will maintain eating the good foods while slowly adding foods you like back and seeing if you have a reaction. That's it. Simple. Going forward you will know what to eat and you will have made life changes to carry you forward into a hopefully very long and healthy life.

To aid this process, I recommend adding bone broth, fermented foods, and a detox drink. While you can still get results without them, I highly (very, very highly) recommend you take the time and effort to add them in. If you are going to make the effort and want results, then do it all and get the best results you can.

Bone Broth

Bone broth sounds weird, but just think of it as the stock for soup. That is basically what it is. It is just cooking bones with marrow in them to pull out minerals and nutrients. It has a high calcium, magnesium, and phosphorous content which is why homemade chicken soup was always associated with helping recover from a cold or flu. It also supports joints, skin, hair, and nails due to the high collagen content.

You make it by first getting some organic bones. If you can't find them in your store, try an Asian grocery, or a local meat store. Beef, chicken, and turkey are the easiest to find. Marrow filled are best because of the dense nutrients. You can also look for left-over parts such as spine, rib cage, chicken feet, or fish heads. Don't worry, you can strain it out if you don't want to eat that part. It can be raw or cooked, so the next time you take apart a chicken or turkey, throw the bones in the pot and start boiling.

I like using a slow cooker, but a soup pot on the stove works just as well.

1. Put the bones in the pot and cover with water.
2. Add a couple tablespoons of apple cider vinegar or lemon juice and let it sit for about 30 minutes. The acid starts the breakdown of the bones into minerals.
3. Bring water to a boil, then cover and reduce to a simmer.
4. Simmer a minimum 6-8 hours for poultry, 4-6 hours for fish, or 12-18 for other types of bones. I prefer the slow cooker where it simmers on low for 24-48 hours.
5. Make sure to add water if necessary. Your lid should be tight enough that steam isn't released, but if not then add water.
6. Salt to taste. If you plan to just drink the broth, salt enhances the flavor and if you use it to cook with, then it would be seasoned anyway.
7. Vegetable remnants can also be added for additional nutrients and flavoring. A stick of celery works well.
8. You can now strain it to make soup, or bottle it if you just want the broth for drinking.
9. Do not skim the fat off when it cools for storage, that part contains nutrients as well. It can be stored in the refrigerator for a week or so or frozen for later.

Bonus: if you have pets, they will love eating the bones you strain out. They should crumble easily so can be safely digested. Add a little broth to their water when they don't feel well and they will lap it up. If you add vegetables or seasonings when making broth, be sure you do not include onions, garlic, chives, peppers including ground, or too much salt. Those can harm your pets. Check before adding anything.

I love making bone broth into a vegetable soup to eat in the morning. It makes it easy to get both the daily broth and your morning veggies eaten. Once you get over the weirdness of soup for breakfast, it is really good.

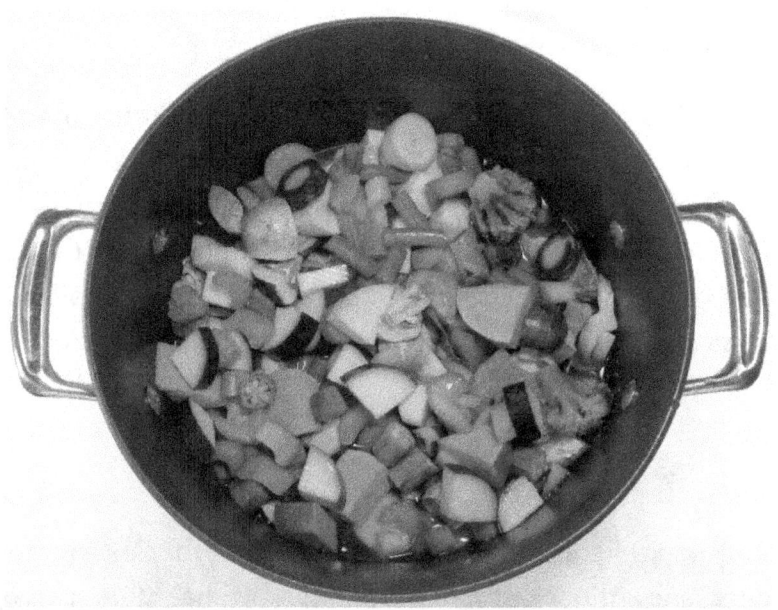

My Bone Broth Vegetable Soup
1. Get a large soup pot.
2. Fill up with all kinds of vegetables including fresh or frozen. If I have it, I throw it in until the pot is almost full.
3. Add bone broth until you can just start seeing the liquid under the veggies.

4. Add salt, pepper, and any spice you like. Turmeric is good, but will stain everything it touches.
5. Cover and simmer on medium/low about 30 minutes. Don't cook vegetables higher as the heat destroys nutrients.
6. Put in jars and you have at least one easy meal a day. I put it in the quart Ball jars, so it is a bowl each for two. One large pot will give me 7 jars, so I have breakfast for a week.

Fermented Foods

For those of us on the American diet, the sound of fermented foods is a bit disgusting. However, it you just think of it as your probiotics in food form, then ah yes, that sounds ok. Sauerkraut, Kimchi, Tempeh, Natto, and Miso are all very good fermented foods. However homemade pickles (not your processed ones), raw cheese, organic salsa, and organic yogurt are also excellent sources.

Detox Drink

This drink is excellent. It includes cranberry juice for clearing stomach disorders and urinary tract infections. It has tart cherry for antioxidants and reduction of pain and inflammation. It has lemon juice for healing vitamin C, flavonoids, and stimulating gastric juices. It also has apple cider vinegar for lowering blood sugar levels and helping you feel fuller. If you are wondering about the sugar in fruit juice, don't worry. These have no sugar added, only natural fructose which is metabolized differently. You will be drinking small amounts and the benefits are tremendous.

Mixture (makes 3 servings):

1. 4 oz. organic 100% pure cranberry juice (not cranberry drink)
2. 2 oz. organic 100% pure tart cherry juice (not cherry drink)
3. 2 tbs. organic 100% pure lemon juice (not lemonade)
4. 1 tsp. organic apple cider vinegar
5. Water down to taste, about 2 parts water to 1-part mixture works well.
6. Drink before meals.

These measurements do not have to be exact. I premix it in the juice jars they come in then add to water and drink daily. I pour half the cranberry juice into another container, pour in the tart cherry until about ¾ full, pour in lemon juice filling half of the left over space, then pour in a good helping of apple cider vinegar. Then I just rinse that jar out when done and use it to make the next batch. This stores well in the refrigerator. Remember however, that this is condensed so you will want to add water before drinking. Measure about 2 oz. of the mixture into your glass and remember it so you don't have to measure every day. Then just add about twice (4 oz.) that amount of cold water and drink. It is very strong tasting, but once you get used to the taste you will learn to really like it.

Vegetables Allowed

You can have unlimited vegetables. Except for a few specific ones, you can eat as much as you want.

Let's make this simple. Vegetables are all grown, so if it is fresh in the produce section or frozen with nothing added, you can have it. Yes, there are choices that are better than others such as sweet potato vs. white potato, or broccoli vs. corn. However, the point is to eat natural foods rather than processed, so eat the best you can. Of course, you need to avoid certain ones during the specific weeks you are detoxing those certain foods, such as white potatoes or corn, but the principle applies to all produce choices.

Organic is the preferred choice for most items because they use organic pesticides and are non GMO. Getting the certification to be sold as organic is expensive though, so the cost is much greater. If you can shop your local farmer's markets, then you can ask and get better and fresher products. If that is not a choice, then you can use the clean/dirty list (see below) to tell which foods you need to be more concerned with. If it is on the dirty list, then try to at least buy those items organic.

There are other factors as well. Foods that are diuretic stimulate urine output and can aid pushing toxins out. This will also reduce fluid swelling, but while some is good, too much can be a problem. Sprinkle a few into your daily intake, but don't just pull from that list.

Nightshades are foods to avoid if you have arthritis or migraines. While they are not definitively linked, a sensitivity to them may bring on those symptoms. Since we are trying to find out what works for you, it is simply easier to avoid them during the detox. You can add them later and see if they have any effect on you.

Additional considerations are whether they are high in starches or where they are grown. Make the best choices from what is available to you. I am of the opinion that if it is natural and doesn't affect you specifically then the nutrients derived outweigh other factors. One being that a sweet potato may be starchy, but it fills me up so I won't hit the vending machine for a snack later. Too many starches will reduce weight loss if that is a goal, so factor that in as you see fit.

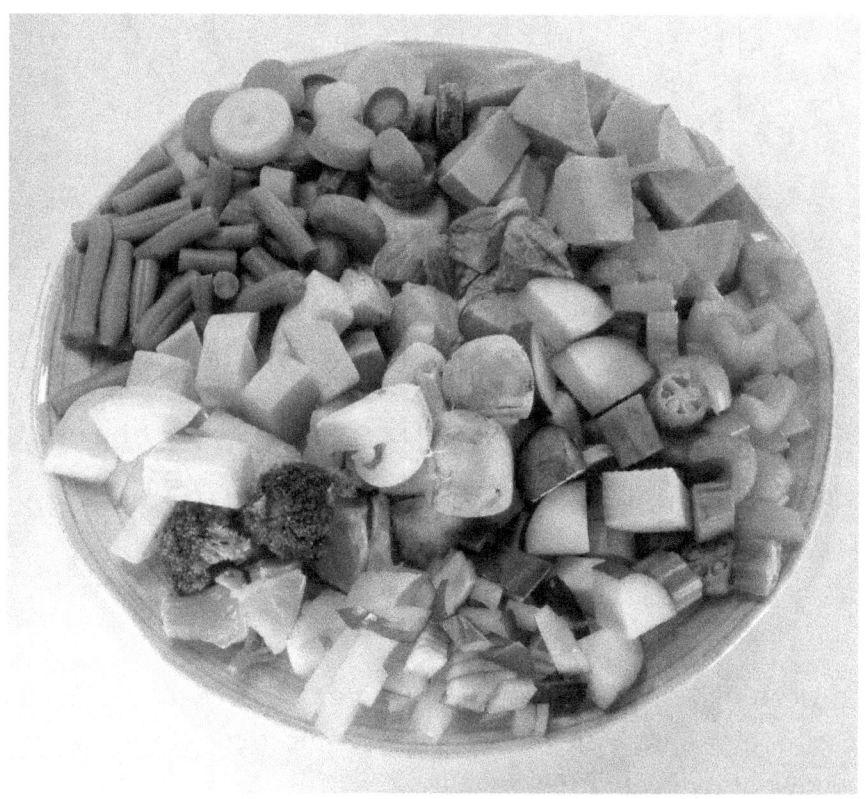

Note: Those items greyed out in the chart below are to be avoided during certain detox weeks.

Clean Fifteen	Dirty Dozen
Avocados	Strawberries
Pineapples	Apples
Cabbage	Nectarines
Onions	Peaches
Asparagus	Celery
Mangos	Grapes
Papayas	Cherries
Kiwi	Spinach
Honeydew Melon	Sweet bell peppers
Grapefruit	Cucumbers
Cantaloupe	Kale/Collard greens
Cauliflower	Hot Peppers
Sweet Peas Frozen	Tomatoes
Sweet Potatoes	Cherry Tomatoes
Sweet Corn	
Eggplant	

The clean and dirty lists are from Environmental Working Group's website, ewg.org. Visit them to get the most current list or more about what is in your food.

Diuretic	Nightshades
Asparagus	Bell/Sweet Peppers
Beets	Potatoes (not Sweet)
Blueberries	Tomatoes
Brussel sprouts	Eggplant
Cabbage	Hot Peppers
Celery	Paprika
Cucumbers	Red Chile Flakes
Garlic	Cayenne
Green tea	
Horseradish	
Lemons	
Leafy greens	
Onions	
Parsley	
Peaches	
Pineapples	
Pears	
Radishes	
Watermelon	
Tomatoes	
Eggplant	

What Not to Eat

You are probably wondering what all you have to give up, well you don't have to give up anything except what is listed for each week. Then once you detox from that food, you will not eat it again until you start reintroducing them in week 8. If you like meat, then eat meat (except the week you detox it). However, try to choose lean and even organic if you can. As for processed foods, these are specifically detoxed in week 4 so before that you can have them (although not recommended). Nuts are not detoxed, so they make excellent snacks at any point. Remember, peanuts are legumes not nuts.

If you don't already eat a lot of vegetables, then adding them should fill you up more. Then you will simply be too full for much else. You will also start feeling better and the cravings should decrease naturally. You can make better choices, and you know what they are, but it is not required to achieve results.

But I Don't Cook

If you don't cook, this is going to be hard. I didn't cook at all before and had to learn while going through this. I still overcook vegetables, but I feel so much better eating healthy than when I go back to bad habits. I now rely on what I call My Vegetable Bake or Hash, but I hope to expand my repertoire in the future.

My Vegetable Bake

1. Preheat oven 400°F.
2. Chop your vegetables into large chunks. (I like yellow squash, zucchini, and mushrooms the most).
3. Throw on a baking pan.
4. Bake 30 minutes.
5. I don't oil or season them as I like the natural flavors just fine.
6. An easier version is to make "boats", just cut them lengthwise and lay them face down.
7. You can also bake chicken this way, so for two, I just put a couple of chicken thighs on one end of the sheet and fill the rest with vegetables and bake the same way. I will add salt and pepper or lemon pepper to the chicken to give it more flavor.

Hash

1. Heat a little oil or butter in a skillet on medium.
2. Add chopped onions, garlic, or whatever you like that takes a little longer to cook.
3. Toss in chopped veggies of whatever is around.
4. Maybe toss in some leftover cooked meat.
5. Season to taste.
6. Cook for just a few minutes and then it's ready to eat.

Notes

- 1 serving of vegetables equals ½ cup or 1 cup loose leaves. Vegetables can be raw or lightly cooked.
- Condiments may contain sugar, so make good choices.
- Salt, pepper, and other spices are not only allowed, but encouraged. They make veggies taste better and add other nutrients on their own.
- Real butter, ghee, olive oil, sesame oil, avocado oil, coconut oil, and grapeseed oil are all fine.
- Salad dressings are ok if they do not contain sugar.
- No, ketchup is not allowed. Homemade would normally be ok, but we are also detoxing tomatoes, so you are out of luck.

The Simplified Program

Starting

Test your results by writing down your starting point.

1. Make a comprehensive list of your current symptoms and rate how much they bother you from 1 to 10. Be sure to include all pains, rashes, hair loss, acne, or things you have lived with for years that have just become a part of your life.
2. Write down your weight and any body measurements you want. (Hint: measure your waist with a string and mark where it meets. Numbers can be depressing, but seeing the mark move can cheer up your day.)
3. Find current lab tests or get them done before starting.

At the end of 8 weeks (before foods are added back), repeat the above and compare. Show yourself it was worth it.

Symptoms Rated 1-10

1 = slightly irritating
5 = bothers me and effects my life some
10 = greatly effects my daily living

My Symptoms	Before Program	After 7 weeks	After 14 weeks

How It Works

Step One: Adding

Add vegetables to every meal. Week One add 2 servings per meal. Weeks Two to Ten add 3 servings to every meal. One serving is ½ cup cooked/raw vegetables or one full cup of loose leaf greens.

Add nutritional aids to support toxin removal. Add bone broth, the detox drink, and fermented foods to your daily routine.

You will continue with these additions for the complete 14 weeks.

Step Two: Eliminating

Each week you will eliminate a food group. **Once it is eliminated you will NOT add it back until at least Week Seven.** Weeks 7 to 14 are for food reintroductions and monitoring how each affects you.

Detox Elimination Schedule:

Week One – caffeine
Week Two – sugar and fruit juice
Week Three – grains, gluten and corn
Week Four – white potatoes, eggs, shellfish, tomatoes, soy, dairy, alcohol, legumes, and all processed foods
Week Five – continue detoxing everything eliminated
Week Six – meat (seafood optional)
Week Seven – reintroduce meat
Weeks Eight-Fourteen – reintroduce other foods slowly (one new food of your choice no closer than every three days)

Week One

Detox Caffeine

If you are a caffeine junky, do **NOT** go cold turkey. Take the time to wean yourself off over several days. If you need to do this more slowly, just take an extra week for this step. This will allow your body to settle down before the next step. It will increase your chances of sticking to the program if you do what is best for your own situation and not try to force the change in a specific amount of time. Caffeine headaches can be debilitating. This should show you just how bad it is for you, and that it is truly a chemical addiction.

Foods to add to your normal diet:

You will be adding a **minimum** of vegetables to your food intake unless you already eat them.

Bone broth, detox drink, and fermented foods are also added.

You should already be drinking water, but it is listed because it is critical to flushing toxins.

Week 1
Detox caffeine

6 servings vegetables (serving = 1/2 cup or 1 cup if loose leaf)
3 servings detox drink (serving = 2 oz. + 4 oz. water)
4 oz. bone broth (1/2 cup)
1 tsp. fermented food
4 servings water (serving = 8 oz. or 1 cup)

Breakfast, Lunch, and Dinner	Detox drink (before)
	2 servings of veggies
	8 oz. water
Any Time	Fermented Food
	Bone Broth
	8 oz. water

Week Two

Detox Sugar and Fruit Juice

Sugar also takes a while to get out of your system. It is highly addictive and the more you have in your diet, the harder it will be to stop eating it. You may experience brain fog, irritability, headaches, and severe cravings for a few days. As your body changes its source of energy from sugar/glucose to tapping fat storage, you may feel fatigued and lethargic. Don't let this stop you. It only proves that you really need to do this.

On the positive side, by the end of the week all those vegetables will taste so much better. Your palate will change and all natural foods will taste sweeter on their own. By the end, you will also feel more energetic, more focused, and happier.

Note: The fruit juices in the detox drink are exceptions. They are specific juices and in relatively small amounts that work with the healing objectives of this program.

Week 2
Detox caffeine
Detox sugar and fruit juice
Add 3 more vegetables to each meal from now on

9 servings vegetables (serving = 1/2 cup or 1 cup if loose leaf)
3 servings detox drink (serving = 2 oz. + 4 oz. water)
4 oz. bone broth (1/2 cup)
1 tsp. fermented food
4 servings water (serving = 8 oz. or 1 cup)

Breakfast, Lunch, and Dinner	Detox drink (before)
	3 servings of veggies
	8 oz. water
Any Time	Fermented Food
	Bone Broth
	8 oz. water

Week Three

Detox Grains, Gluten and Corn

If you have severe gastric issues, eliminating these may produce significant changes in how you feel. If you are not sensitive to them, then you won't feel symptom relief, but you may lose weight.

Week 3
Detox caffeine
Detox sugar and fruit juice
Detox grains, gluten and corn

9 servings vegetables (serving = 1/2 cup or 1 cup if loose leaf)
3 servings detox drink (serving = 2 oz. + 4 oz. water)
4 oz. bone broth (1/2 cup)
1 tsp. fermented food
4 servings water (serving = 8 oz. or 1 cup)

Breakfast, Lunch, and Dinner	Detox drink (before)
	3 servings of veggies
	8 oz. water
Any Time	Fermented Food
	Bone Broth
	8 oz. water

Week Four

Detox White Potatoes, Eggs, Shellfish, Tomatoes, Soy, Dairy, Alcohol, Legumes, and All Processed Foods

Common legumes are peanuts, lentils, and all beans. You might wonder why these naturally grown foods are on the list, but it is because they can cause gastric problems for some. Properly cooking them (after soaking, sprouting, or fermenting) reduces this, but as we are eliminating common food allergies, legumes are on the list. Fresh or frozen green beans and green peas are okay because they have never been dried and after cooking have a very low likelihood of causing gastric issues.

Sorry about the alcohol and dairy. Those may be hard, but you can live without them for a few weeks. You just might learn something from how your body reacts to not having them.

Real butter is noted as okay above. While it is dairy, cooking with a small amount should not be an issue as the way it is made makes it less sensitive. You can eliminate it if you want.

Processed foods are the hardest. With all the vegetables you have been eating, you should have already greatly reduced these. This is when you have to buckle down and really start cooking healthy.

Week 4
Detox caffeine
Detox sugar and fruit juice
Detox grains, gluten and corn
Detox white potatoes, eggs, shellfish, tomatoes, soy, dairy, alcohol, legumes, and all processed foods

9 servings vegetables (serving = 1/2 cup or 1 cup if loose leaf)
3 servings detox drink (serving = 2 oz. + 4 oz. water)
4 oz. bone broth (1/2 cup)
1 tsp. fermented food
4 servings water (serving = 8 oz. or 1 cup)

Breakfast, Lunch, and Dinner	Detox drink (before)
	3 servings of veggies
	8 oz. water
Any Time	Fermented Food
	Bone Broth
	8 oz. water

Keep Going, you should only be eating good clean food here.

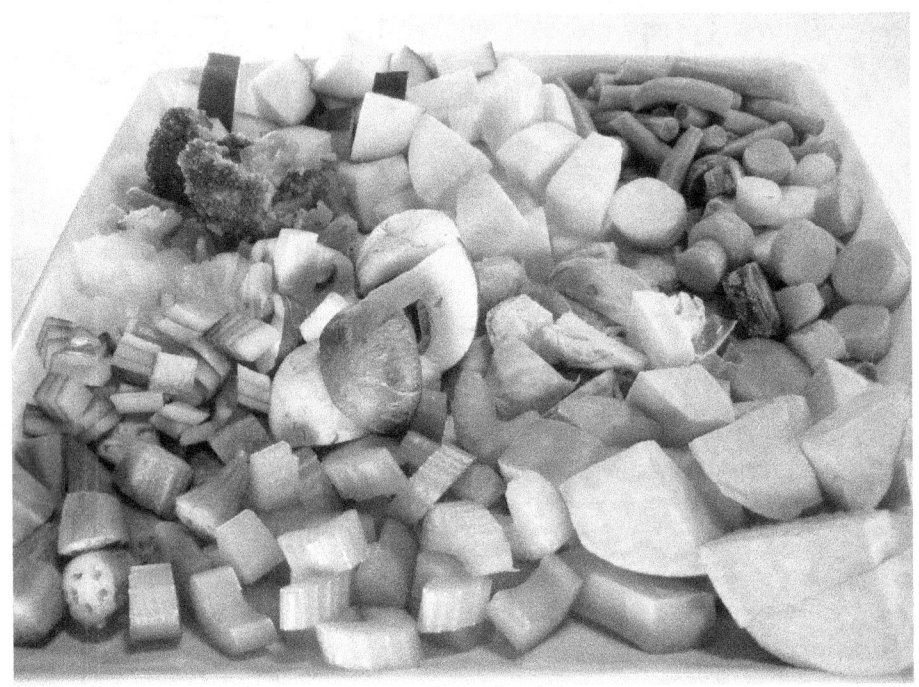

Week 5
Detox caffeine
Detox sugar and fruit juice
Detox grains, gluten and corn
Detox white potatoes, eggs, shellfish, tomatoes, soy, dairy, alcohol, legumes, and all processed foods
No additional foods to eliminate this week

9 servings vegetables (serving = 1/2 cup or 1 cup if loose leaf)
3 servings detox drink (serving = 2 oz. + 4 oz. water)
4 oz. bone broth (1/2 cup)
1 tsp. fermented food
4 servings water (serving = 8 oz. or 1 cup)

Breakfast, Lunch, and Dinner	Detox drink (before)
	3 servings of veggies
	8 oz. water
Any Time	Fermented Food
	Bone Broth
	8 oz. water

Detox Meat

If you are worried about a lack of protein, don't be. Protein is in vegetables, nuts, and seeds. Try some almonds, sunflower seeds, avocado, broccoli, spinach, and kale for good sources.

Most people do not have a sensitivity to lean meats, but it has been known to happen, so we go ahead and eliminate it for this week. It also gives your gut a chance to clear out any undigested meats that may cause stomach issues.

You have an option here to include seafood in the detox. Poultry, red meats, and pork are the main culprits you need to eliminate, so if you want to continue eating seafood you can. If you think seafood may be an issue based on how your body reacts, then eliminate it too. Seafood contain their own toxins such as mercury that are good to flush, but you can always eliminate them later if you still have symptoms you are trying to pin down.

Week 6
Detox caffeine
Detox sugar and fruit juice
Detox grains, gluten and corn
Detox white potatoes, eggs, shellfish, tomatoes, soy, dairy, alcohol, legumes, and all processed foods
Detox meat (seafood optional)

9 servings vegetables (serving = 1/2 cup or 1 cup if loose leaf)
3 servings detox drink (serving = 2 oz. + 4 oz. water)
4 oz. bone broth (1/2 cup)
1 tsp. fermented food
4 servings water (serving = 8 oz. or 1 cup)

Breakfast, Lunch, and Dinner	Detox drink (before)
	3 servings of veggies
	8 oz. water
Any Time	Fermented Food
	Bone Broth
	8 oz. water

Week Seven

Keep Going

You can reintroduce meat this week, but if you want to continue longer without, then by all means, continue without. If you do reintroduce it, make sure it is lean and preferably organic or locally sourced.

Week 7
Detox caffeine
Detox sugar and fruit juice
Detox grains, gluten and corn
Detox white potatoes, eggs, shellfish, tomatoes, soy, dairy, alcohol, legumes, and all processed foods
Reintroduce meat

9 servings vegetables (serving = 1/2 cup or 1 cup if loose leaf)
3 servings detox drink (serving = 2 oz. + 4 oz. water)
4 oz. bone broth (1/2 cup)
1 tsp. fermented food
4 servings water (serving = 8 oz. or 1 cup)

Breakfast, Lunch, and Dinner	Detox drink (before)
	3 servings of veggies
	8 oz. water
Any Time	Fermented Food
	Bone Broth
	8 oz. water

Weeks Eight to Fourteen

Remaining Food Reintroduction

For the next few weeks you will be reintroducing foods to your system. You can add one type of food every three days. You need to pay attention here, because if you have a sensitivity to that food, you should notice fairly quickly.

At the start of week 8, you will want to write another comprehensive symptom list. Compare it to the one you did before you started this program and see what's changed. You should have eliminated a lot of your daily issues. If not, you may want to evaluate what you are still eating and try eliminating more.

Consider any oils you are cooking with, or specific vegetables you are eating.

FODMAPs can also cause gastric issues. These include garlic and onions, which many of us use for flavoring, as well as many other vegetables. They are short-chain carbohydrates that that do not get completely absorbed in the intestinal tract leaving sugars that feed bad gut flora or ferment in the gut. This causes gas, pain, and diarrhea.

You may also be getting small amounts of something you are sensitive to through other sources you are unaware of. Many supplements contain gluten, corn, or dairy so if you are highly sensitive, this may affect you. Salad dressings also have lots of unexpected ingredients. This is where you need to put on your investigation cap and narrow it down. Don't forget about things like nickel in a cooking pans or plastics in your containers. Make sure you have good tools to cook your good food with.

If you are taking medications, pay close attention to how you feel. Your body chemistry has altered now so you may want to see your doctor and redo any necessary lab tests.

Weeks 8-14
Begin reintroduction of remaining detoxed foods one at a time. Do not add more than one every three days. Watch for reactions.

9 servings vegetables (serving = 1/2 cup or 1 cup if loose leaf)
3 servings detox drink (serving = 2 oz. + 4 oz. water)
4 oz. bone broth (1/2 cup)
1 tsp. fermented food
4 servings water (serving = 8 oz. or 1 cup)

Breakfast, Lunch, and Dinner	Detox drink (before)
	3 servings of veggies
	8 oz. water
Any Time	Fermented Food
	Bone Broth
	8 oz. water

After the Detox

Eating this many vegetables a day and making sure you consume enough water are practices you should now live with daily. This is just eating healthy. While you may not want bone broth and fermented foods every day, eating them regularly will provide huge benefits. They are your minerals and probiotics, which added to the vitamins in vegetables, proteins in lean meats, and healthy fats in healthy oils you have all of your required nutrients.

The detox drink is good to have occasionally, especially if you need to clear your system from a binge or a wild holiday where you ate anything and everything.

This program is simply another tool in your tool box for a healthy life. If you revert to old habits or just feel generally toxic, come back and start this program again. If you have learned which foods you are ok with, then you might not need to eliminate them again. Use the basics but modify it to work for you.

Going Forward
Continue these practices as much as you are able.

6-9 servings vegetables (serving = 1/2 cup or 1 cup if loose leaf)
3 servings detox drink (serving = 2 oz. + 4 oz. water)
4 oz. bone broth (1/2 cup)
1 tsp. fermented food
4 servings water (serving = 8 oz. or 1 cup)

Breakfast, Lunch, and Dinner	Detox drink (before)
	2-3 servings of veggies
	8 oz. water
Any Time	Fermented Food
	Bone Broth
	8 oz. water

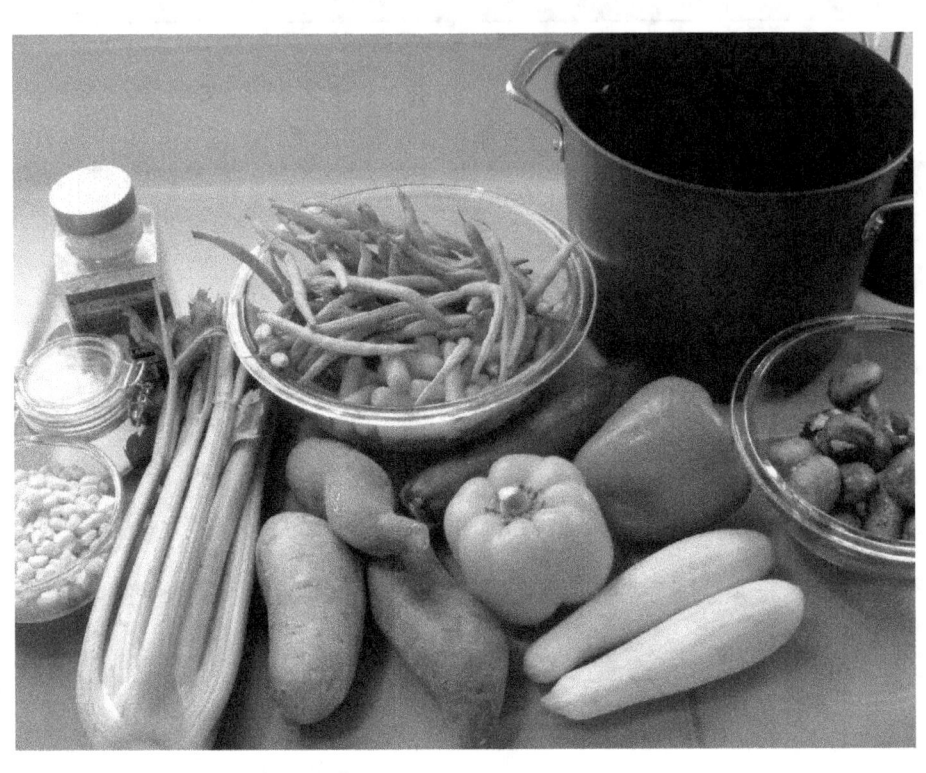

I hope you were able to complete the program as closely as possible the first time and you had positive results. Thanks and here's wishing you a happy and healthy life forward.

Be well and live healthy!

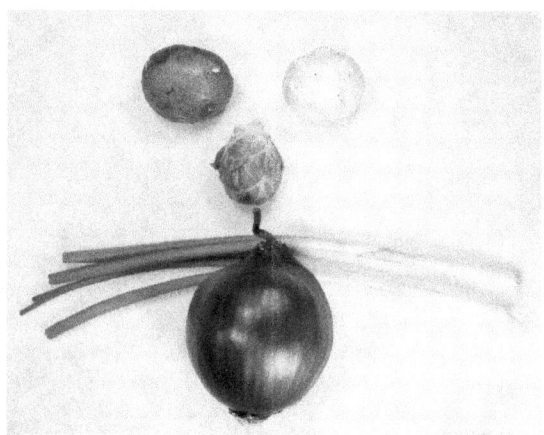

About the Author

Hello everyone. So about me. I became a Chiropractor because I was interested in alternative healing practices. Like so many others, I was drawn to it because of health issues of my own or my family. I wasn't getting answers or solutions after a couple of years of doctors, so I started studying on my own. When I learned that Chiropractic was about healing the whole body rather than eliminating symptoms, I was hooked. While manual adjustments are the basis of Chiropractic, the philosophy of whole body healing must include nutritional support. Making it simple for patients is my goal and the reason I put this book together. I wanted to eliminate the extra hundred or so pages of science behind the reasons for each step of this program and just boil it down to what steps to take. I hope those who complete the program not only have extremely positive results, but also learn about the relationship of food and daily wellness.

Find other useful tips on my website **Nutri4m.com.**

A review of this book would be appreciated and watch for my next book to come out soon!